MEDICAL SCHOOL, NOW WHAT?: A GUIDE TO BUILDING A REWARDING PRACTICE

GARY D. STEINMAN, MD, PhD

WITH TECHNICAL ASSISTANCE IN PART FROM:

ALAN R. POLLACK, ESQ.

AND

DAVID L. SCHWARTZ, CPA

BAFFIN PUBLISHING COMPANY

NEW YORK, NY

2011

Medical School, Now What? A Guide to

Building a Rewarding Practice

by Gary D. Steinman, MD, PhD

Published by: Baffin Publishing Company

19918 Epsom Course, Holliswood, New York 11423

E-mail: BAFFINPUBLISHING@gmail.com

Website: www.baffinpublishing.com

Copyright © 2011 by Gary D. Steinman

First printing – 2011   Printed by: BookMasters, Inc.

Printed in United States   Cover design: Kim Casteel

Title creator: Mike Erickson

Library of Congress Control Number: 2011908177

ISBN: 978-0-9665105-2-2

    I.   Medicine-Practice.

    II.   Physicians-finance, personal

Previous books by Gary Steinman:

Biochemical Predestination, 1969

Doctor-to-Doctor: Avoiding Financial Suicide, 1998

Womb Mates – a Modern Guide to Fertility and Twinning, 2007

ב"ה

This book is dedicated to *my* magnificent seven:

Jessica,

Allegra,

Ahuvah,

Jeremiah,

Zechariah,

Moriah,

Batsheva

INTRODUCTION

In a study recently published in *Academic Medicine*, medical students expressed general satisfaction with their training in patient care. In contradistinction, less than half felt they had received adequate instruction in practice management and medical economics. From the inception of a practice, attention must be given to the proper management of funds needed to cover all expenses, personal or professional, planned or unanticipated. **In spite of advanced education, doctors are infamous for their general lack of knowledge in medical economics.**

This book is written with the assumption that the *student doctor* (medical student; resident) will enter practice upon completing his training. Most new physicians today are joining group or hospital-based practices. Some discussion specifically directed to negotiating contracts with group employers is included. The same principles that are intended for the solo practitioner apply equally to doctors employed by hospitals and group practices. Similarly, *doctors already in practice* can improve their organization with the information provided here.

In much the same way that a well-trained physician actively manages the medical situations under his care, so too, he should be prepared to manage his own financial and economic health. If the reader is now a medical student or a resident, he/she has already defined in his/her mind why each wants to be a doctor. Medicine is not just a way to earn a living; it is also an expression of one's empathy for sick people and desire to do something to make their lives healthier. It is a unique profession which has an immense impact on the people served. **A well-run, well-organized medical practice can be rewarding for the doctor in at least two ways: professionally and economically.**

The subjects that follow were carefully selected by and from the perspective of a practicing physician to be among those about which every doctor should have a working knowledge and understanding *before* he completes his formal training. (Most medical schools do not yet provide formal instruction in this important area of professional activity.) This book is designed as a guide to basic subjects and as a handy reference for orientation into areas of particular interest to the practitioner. It is not intended to be an encyclopedic source of information.

Medical economics is no less complex than neuroanatomy or molecular biology. The topics discussed in this book are not overly simplified since a broad understanding of them is necessary to setting up and maintaining an efficient, productive medical practice.

The discussions to be considered here are written in terminology comprehensible to the non-economist (e.g., physician). The methods suggested for managing financial matters are condensed and summarized into formats which should be understandable to the general public. By no means are the explanations meant to be exhaustive and technically thorough. Through insights into the mechanisms of economic activities, the medical practitioner should gain perspective as to how one develops and sustains financial security. Each subject is presented as an *introduction* to the salient features of a fundamental definition, concept, or function.

In the same way that physicians update their professional skills through their continuing medical education, the student/doctor/spouse/parent must continue to sharpen his/her knowledge in the economic realm throughout life to effectively serve his key responsibilities within the personal sphere as well. Just as providers work (or will work) hard to earn the money from a practice in the first place, each must also formulate a modus operandi to make the proceeds perform effectively for him to enhance his future economic health. This requires knowledgeable planning and execution of an investment program under the practitioner's primary control.

The terms "doctor" and "physician" used in this text embrace all healthcare providers (HCP), including dentists, osteopathic physicians, speech pathologists, optometrists, podiatrists, MDs, physical therapists, veterinarians, nurse practitioners, chiropractors, psychologists, radiotherapists, audiologists, physiologists, rehabilitation therapists, nutritionists, pharmacists, hospitalists, medical students, interns, residents, etc.

The generic terms "he" and "his" applied here should be taken to refer equally to female and male physicians, single or married, throughout this book. The financial issues to be raised here apply in the same way to both genders.

Statistics show that more women are entering medicine today than ever before, now representing about ⅓ of all graduate physicians in the US. Whereas the number of women in American medical schools in 1961 was 6% of the student body, by 2006 this number had risen to 49%. Unfortunately, in a recent study it was reported that women physicians earn 39% less than their male counterparts, for various reasons (including time-out for child-rearing).

The subjects to be covered here include:

- PRACTICE – choosing between solo and group; selecting a specialty.

- MANAGEMENT – organized, effective business procedures to safeguard orderly growth of a practice.

- INSURANCE – imperative key programs early in a practice to secure an instant estate and a stable financial future.

- BUDGETING – effective control of personal expenditures to avoid expansion of debt beyond serviceable levels.

- PENSION – deferring income for future needs and for tax savings must begin with the startup of any practice (including joining a group).

- INVESTMENTS – self-directed growth of savings to promote a continuous increase in net worth and standard of living.

- ASSET PROTECTION – with the specter of malpractice, divorce, and health problems forever looming, one must shield his finances _early_ to protect them from potential future assault.

- ETHICS – compassionate care

SPECIAL NOTICE

In no way is this book intended to function as an exhaustive, detailed legal reference or primary source. Before making vital financial decisions, the reader must consult with proper experts and authoritative sources for more complete, definitive explanations and advice as needed. With time and experience, the doctor will gain confidence and insight, and will be able to assume greater primary responsibility for the investment decisions in his portfolio.

This book is designed to provide an introductory overview of applicable information in the subject matter covered. It is sold with the understanding that the author and the publisher are not engaged in the profession of rendering legal, accounting, investment, insurance, or other financial services.

Every effort has been devoted to make this book as thorough, concise, and accurate as possible. Errors related to typographical and technical matters may have entered the manuscript unintentionally. The most up-to-date legal rulings, legislations, tax laws, and opinions should be obtained from appropriate professional experts. This educational text should only be used as a general guide and not as an ultimate source for making financial decisions.

The author of this book is not a Certified Financial Planner or a graduate lawyer; therefore, the author, consultants, and publisher of this book shall have neither liability nor responsibility to any person or entity with respect to any loss or damage caused, or alleged to be caused, directly or indirectly, by the information contained in the book. If the purchaser does not wish to be bound by these limitations and precautions, the book may returned this book in resalable condition to the publisher or his distributor for a full refund.

ABOUT THE AUTHOR

Dr. Steinman began his professional career studying for his doctorate in biophysics at the University of California, Berkeley, under Nobel Prize winner Prof. Melvin Calvin. After co-authoring the book, *Biochemical Predestination,* on the origin of life on Earth, Dr. Steinman responded to a call from NASA for applicants to the Scientist-Astronaut Program. Though he qualified for the program, he elected to pursue other interests, including the position of Managing Director of a science-based company in Israel. This was followed by a medical degree from the University of Miami and then an office and hospital-based career in Obstetrics and Gynecology. He subsequently wrote *Doctor-to-Doctor: Avoiding financial suicide*, the forerunner to the present book.

The author is now Chairman of Biochemistry at Touro College of Osteopathic Medicine in New York and Assistant Clinical Professor at Albert Einstein School of Medicine. His research interest is in twinning and he has appeared on *National Geographic TV*, among others, discussing this subject. He has lectured internationally and recently published the book, *Womb Mates – A Modern Guide to Fertility and Twinning.*

Dr. Steinman has seven children and lives in New York. Outside of work, he enjoys dogsledding in the Arctic (see back cover).

TABLE OF CONTENTS

Chapter 1 - Basic Economic and Professional Goals

Just as he must prudently select consultants to assist in the resolution of a medical problem with his patients, the doctor should wisely choose knowledgeable, objective financial advisers (see Chap.7) to provide applicable opinions and suggestions; however, it is the physician himself who must ultimately elect the final approach to take, and be prepared to modify that approach depending on how events unfold.

From the inception of a practice, attention must be given to funds needed to cover equipment, salaries, insurance and rent. A modest beginning can be embellished as patient load and income increase. Even if one's father were Bill Gates or Nelson Rockefeller, it is the practitioner's responsibility to generate income from his practice and his investments to support himself and his family.

The student doctor must absorb an immense volume of material to prepare him for independent clinical work. As a result, unfortunately, he is typically unversed in the special knowledge needed to effectively control and direct his own financial future. Most new physicians following residency (and many seasoned practitioners, for that matter) do not have an understanding of issues related to disciplined spending, effective business practices, and wise investing in the real world. The possession of a medical degree alone is no longer a guarantee of lifetime wealth.

For philosophical reasons, doctors may feel that attention to monetary issues taints their professional stature and their perceived dedication to helping people, until the accounts payable (money owed by the doctor for supplies, insurance, salaries, etc.) start coming due. In fact, the converse is true; namely, a well-run business office can better serve the community of patients seeking healthcare services there. This is not being mercenary; it is being realistic.

The managed care revolution and the rapid rise in medical malpractice insurance premiums have diminished the income expectations of the healthcare provider; however, the professional who has struggled through medical training for the purpose of aiding people is no less a dedicated, ethical, or effective as a physician if his financial life is properly arranged and in order. A doctor is entitled to be compensated for his time and expertise, just as the merchant should be paid for the computer he sells him to run his practice.

With the prestige and money which medical practice imparts, the typical doctor is mesmerized by the expectation that he may well attain a net worth in excess of $1,000,000 during his career; however, because of disregard and indifference in his early professional years, he might not prepare for the needs of later years. Funds are consumed with luxuries; delinquent accounts receivable (money due the doctor for his services) are ignored too easily because of ineffective bookkeeping.

Essential instruments which should be implemented early on, to set the stage for immediate and future financial security for himself and his dependents, are not initiated. These include life insurance, children's educational savings, and pension, among others. They are put off to a later date when it may, in fact, leave insufficient time for adequate accumulation and effective protection.

In essence, the adage "you work 30 years to live 60 years" is not fully appreciated in many cases until it is too late. **The typical physician spends about half his adult life without earning income from his profession** (in school and, later, in retirement).

Newly graduated doctors are prime targets for lenders who are anxious to extend credit to professionals with the acknowledged potential for strong future earnings. For the young practitioner, it is an over-whelming temptation to "buy now and pay later," with new debt (especially high-interest-rate credit cards) added on to outstanding educational loans. Borrowing to invest in items needed to initiate and promote a practice is one thing; untimely personal extravagance is another. In this way, much of his career is a struggle to meet repayment demands and postpone more important issues, such as pension and diversified savings "for a rainy day." Credit ratings suffer as a result. Many doctors reach their 50s and begin to consider slowing down and even retiring, only to find that they must continue working hard for several more years just to "make ends meet." Many very successful practices are tragically reduced to bankruptcy because of inadequate planning and imprudent spending.

This book presents an ***introduction*** to key concepts and terms which are vital for the doctor to understand so that he may map out an appropriate strategy from day #1. It is assumed that the typical reader has little or no prior experience with money management, other than balancing a checking account. Most doctors think they know everything about everything, but sooner or later come to the realization that this is not true in many areas of knowledge, especially financial matters. This book is designed to give the healthcare provider insight into this important realm of life so that germane subjects can be considered and acted upon.

Only the individual himself can truly care enough about his own professional, financial, and personal life to maximize reasonable earnings. He must not assign to others the responsibility for making major decisions because of the fear of a mistake or the assumption that he does not know (or care to know) enough about the subject to act wisely, effectively and ***independently***. Just as the good parent would not delegate to others the major decisions regarding how his/her children are raised, so too, must the provider learn how to take an active role in making prudent economic decisions for the family. It is perplexing to observe how professionals who are trained to act decisively in life-threatening emergency medical situations dodge the prospect of dealing with their own financial matters.

Most conscientious advisers, lawyers, business managers, insurance agents and accountants endeavor to help the doctor satisfy his financial needs through the application of their know-how from _their_ perspective. It is, however, in the end the doctor alone who must decide if any particular advice is really in _his_ best interest. He should not rely on the trite adage healthcare providers traditionally used with their patients: "Trust me; I know what is best for you."

The patient population today is more discerning and now demands informed disclosures. Likewise, the doctor must knowledgeably comprehend **all** the details of the plans being proposed for his and his family's financial health before he consents to them. He must take command and be on top of all activities within and outside his practice, without relinquishing the authority over key decisions and functions to others.

Contrary to popular belief, physicians do <u>not</u> have unlimited earning potential. Managed care appeared when it became apparent that money available for medical care is not limitless. Similarly, the physician needs to understand that his money is not boundless either. He must learn how to administer his expenditures knowledgeably and insightfully for maximum benefit. Foregoing extravagance in the early years of a practice reduces tension which accompanies concern for debt repayment.

In the early years of practice, he may have to forgo the big car, the big house and the big vacations even if lenders are willing to provide the capital to meet these dreams. Investment for basic professional equipment is one thing, but splurging on deferrable personal luxuries is another. It is the long term that must be at the forefront of every doctor's game plan. Recent medical graduates do not *"deserve"* these extravagant treats because they worked hard to get there, any more than any other working person does, until they are able to methodically resolve the more critical basic issues first (e.g., food and housing). Worry about potential or actual excess debt is disconcerting.

A car will only travel as far as the gasoline put into it will allow. Similarly, each person should limit his present spending to his currently available cash (in excess of that needed to meet present basic needs), and funds he can reasonably expect to have accessible soon, without sacrificing safety and security in the near or long term. This requires discipline, self-control and maturity.

Sensible planning should mean a slow, steady, lifelong growth of net worth, rather than a fling at making a quick "killing" with high risk investments. (The Brooklyn Bridge is not for sale!) This approach results in a gradual rise in one's standard of living, rather than an abrupt change which acutely swells debt obligations. ***Deficit spending*** may be standard operating procedure for governments but can be disastrous for individuals.

For most people, it is difficult to contemplate their own mortality or potential for disability, especially during the youthful, healthful years. Young doctors think that only their patients get sick. However, doctors are real people too, and they must confront the possibility of these needs arising earlier than they may have hoped for or anticipated. The author knows of more than one case of a promising medical student/resident who developed a disabling condition and became a patient instead of a provider for an extended period of time. His/her progress in the profession had to be put on hold indefinitely.

"The only two things guaranteed in life are death and taxes."   Benjamin Franklin

"The only certainty in life is change."

Henry A. Wallace

Nothing should be taken for granted. Thus, early planning is vital. Family security is at stake.

Soon after the moment of birth, each individual is faced with an increasing array of personal and environmental *decisions*. This may start with selecting with which toy to play, advancing to food choices, and later what career path to pursue. With increasing age and the assumption of new responsibilities, the methods for providing for one's own needs and, eventually, those of one's dependents become an escalating concern for each person.

Central to this are earning a living and ***supporting a family***. Entering the practice of medicine is no guarantee of a life of ease ensuing from the haphazard management of one's assets. First comes the hard-won attainment of monetary gain from a medical practice. Most people who enter this profession do so (or at least say they do) to provide compassionate care for the sick. As a reward for several years of unpaid (or underpaid) effort to acquire this knowledge, they now can expect a return for their monetary and temporal investment once a practice is embarked upon.

Occupations are roughly divided into two categories: those that yield a *product* and others that provide a *service*. The practice of medicine falls within the second category. Doctors are reimbursed for the time and knowhow they devote to each patient to resolve a medical situation.

Learning to hit a home run requires practice and insight. Whereas a professional baseball player may earn much more *per hour* of work, the doctor has the added satisfaction of using his/her knowledge to reduce human suffering as well. Just as the ball player expects compensation for the energy and skill applied to his trade, so too, the doctor should anticipate a financial return for past and present efforts.

From the standpoint of *earning a living*, there is much in common between the ball player and the physician. Each has a responsibility to himself and his dependents now and in the future. Earning capacity now has applications currently to provide for his family as well as later in his senior years when he may no longer be practicing his profession. In the latter phase, that for which he planned and saved previously becomes crucially important for sustaining his existence into the *retirement* years.

Young doctors give little thought to anticipating their needs several years down the road. They are disconnected from and disinterested in the reality of their own ultimate aging; however, total entropy change is irreversible in an isolated system and the overall trend of the human experience, without exception, is downhill physically and medically. As will be seen in later chapters, the earlier each plans for needs in his/her more senior years, the more that part of one's life becomes tolerable and sustainable. **True wealth is measured by what one has in**

reserve for future needs, not what has already been spent.

Finally, like any commercial undertaking, the principle of supply-and-demand, as determined by societal needs, has relevance in selecting the field of medicine in which one will practice. For example, given present trends, it is estimated that there will be a shortage of over 45,000 primary care physicians in America by 2020. The supply of such doctors has not kept pace with increased demand for a number of reasons:

a) Following World War II, there was a temporary surge in reproduction in the United States. These "baby boomers" are now reaching retirement age.

b) In 2011, the average age of the population has risen to 36.9 years (compared to 32.9 in 1990), in large part due to a current fertility rate (children/woman by age 45) of 2.1, about equal to the replacement value.

c) New Federal legislation has made a larger segment of the people living in America eligible for healthcare insurance.

d) Building of new medical schools has not kept up with demand, especially during the last two decades of the 20th Century.

e) Life expectancy has risen, largely because of the near total control/elimination of fatal infections. Also, major health problems of aging are delayed due to improved treatments of hypertension, diabetes, cancer, and vascular disease, as well as reduced environmental risks such as smoking. (Obesity and sedentary lifestyle have yet to achieve this level of improvement.) As a result, acute medical problems in young and middle-aged people have been replaced by chronic conditions in the elderly ($\geq$65). By 2030, the elderly are expected to represent about 20% of the total US population.

Thus, in making a **career decision**, it is essential for the doctor-in-training to consider several factors, including personal preferences and interests, financial objectives, and the needs of the community.

In summary, each person's ***economic goals*** can be summarized overall as:

1) Increase net worth currently for present and future needs; and

2) Protect net worth once obtained against potential assault.

Subsequent chapters will discuss in detail the means for achieving these goals. During the training years in particular, it is most appropriate for the student doctor to accumulate the professional and fiscal knowhow needed to meet these objectives and to put into motion the modalities for carrying them out.

BASIC ECONOMIC GOALS

INCREASING NET WORTH
PROTECTING NET WORTH
WORK 30 YEARS TO LIVE 60 YEARS

Chapter 2 – Documents and Decisions to Start Practicing

If the reader is now in his residency, the first day of his new medical practice is quickly approaching. Even though one may be entering a group practice, the issues about to be discussed are, for the most part, necessary for each to understand to remain as clear-headed as possible in dealing with new areas of concern in his profession.

Although certificates of graduation from medical school and residency program are tightly held in each candidate's warm hand, certain other documents are required by the various governmental and professional agencies to practice in a community setting. If there is uncertainty about where to get these documents, calls or emails to the appropriate offices should expedite the resolution of these issues.

1) ***Medical license:*** Early application to the health department of the state in which one intends to practice is essential, with evidence of completion of the necessary training and passing the required licensing exam. This process should be completed during residency so that document is available on practice day #1. This

licensure is subject to periodic renewal. Do not complain about the fee – there is no alternative. **Board certification** in the field of practice elected should be secured and maintained throughout one's professional years.

2) Similarly, a license to prescribe controlled substances must be obtained from the US Drug Enforcement Administration (**DEA**). No one can do this for the doctor. Do not fail to provide all information requested truthfully. These agencies have a long memory and know more about each practitioner than one may want to believe.

It is technically illegal for any doctor to write prescriptions, especially for controlled substances, for friends and family if they are not formally the practitioner's patients. The prescription of all medications is limited to patients with whom the doctor has a patient-physician relationship and a medical record documenting these details. If it involves a controlled substance, the DEA number must be included on the written prescription. Violating this can result in fines and, possibly, the loss of a medical license.

3) It is standard now for the parents of nearly all individuals born in the US to secure a *Social Security* registration and ID card soon after birth. This number will be needed in many personal transactions throughout life. In addition, if the practitioner is to employ assistants, an Employer Identification Number (*EIN*) must be obtained by him for Internal Revenue tax purposes.

A recent innovation has been the assignment of a unique 10-digit identification number for all healthcare providers who serve Medicare and Medicaid recipients. This number (National Provider Identifier – *NPI*) is needed for claims submission. Also, physicians who may want to treat workers injured or disabled on their jobs should register with their state's Worker's Compensation Board.

4) Other than the choice of a spouse and a specialty, the most momentous decision a doctor-to-be must make is the *location* of his

practice. In some cases, physicians elect to return to the town in which they were raised because of its familiarity and preexisting social contacts. Another possibility is to continue in the same hospital in which the residency was completed. In a given community, many doctors decide to open an office in a multi-specialty center since referral of patients from other practices at that facility is more readily effected.

5) At the beginning of the final year of residency, a decision should be made how each doctor would like to continue his/her professional activities (solo, group, hospitalist, subspecialty training, research, teaching). The sooner formal job-hunting begins, the more likely specific goals and objectives will be reached.

a) If the graduate enters solo practice, he/she may start a new office or may take over the practice of a physician about to retire. In terms of taxation, the new entity will be considered a sole proprietorship. To be sure records are being kept correctly and the right tax deductions are made, the help of a CPA is usually essential at the outset (see Chaps. 3 and 7).

b) If one is joining a group or a hospital staff, he will be taxed as an employee and the employer will make the appropriate deductions at source monthly.

c) Locating a position can be expedited by recruiting several sources of help and information:

i) The Chief of Service can identify positions available outside the institution as well as those open with attendings in his department. In addition, the department may be seeking new staff members.

ii) The professional journals in each specialty typically have ads near the end of each issue announcing open positions throughout the US.

iii) Each professional association (e.g., American College of Obstetrics &

Gynecology) typically has offices which help put employers and new graduates together.

iv) Networking is very helpful. Make it known as widely as possible with professional colleagues what the candidate is seeking.

v) "Head hunters" are commercial groups which help active physicians find new members to join their practices. They often advertise in professional journals. The service fee is usually paid by the employer.

6) ***Solo versus group***: If a physician joins a preformed group, initial income is higher than that of a solo practitioner since a ready-made patient population exists, startup costs have been absorbed, and business-related expenses are already covered. In the long-run, however, the potential lifetime earnings may be higher for the solo practitioner, especially since he will usually work more hours/week than a doctor in a group.

A recent graduate might elect to open a new office or may continue an ongoing practice to be left by a retiring physician. A fresh solo practice, in particular, grows based on reputation spread by satisfied patients primarily. This may take as much as five years to reach a good level.

It is generally noted that as the number of doctors in a group increases arithmetically, the size of the support staff increases exponentially. Managerial decision-making becomes more complex as a result. The solo practitioner lives by the policies he alone makes without having to compromise his independence with possibly less worthy ideas. On the other hand, the member of a group is better able to preplan his time away from the practice because of cross-coverage than the doctor in solo practice.

An alternative to the conventional pattern of fee-for-service office practice is the recently developed framework of "*concierge*" medicine, especially for primary care. Patients prepay a single annual fee in exchange for more personalized attention, unlimited visits, and more readily available access to the doctor. Insurance such as Medicare will still cover ancillary matters such as medication, specialist visits, hospitalizations and tests.

A growing trend in American medicine is for individual physicians or groups of physicians to leave private practice and to integrate into the overall service programs of hospitals. They become salaried employees (*hospitalists*) of the organization, and the hospital takes over their administrative and overhead responsibilities. Also, they may become part of a group practice within the institution. This gives the doctor greater latitude for involvement in personal activities outside of the practice (e.g., child-rearing).

A variation of this is to join an *academic* facility fulltime. This would usually include teaching medical students and residents, research, and participation in a clinic practice within the auspices of the medical school or teaching hospital. Another possibility would be working for the Government, a research laboratory, or an industrial organization, but this does not usually include seeing patients.

7) **Negotiating** with a group: The formal conditions and details of a contract one receives with an offer to join a group must be taken very seriously. These stipulations will govern your lifestyle for the months and years to come. Usually, it would be most productive if one joins a group in which he/she will remain for a long time.

In some cases, groups take advantage of a neophyte, and for this reason, *experienced legal advice* must be obtained before formalizing an association. Lawyers proficient in this area are essential at this stage before finalizing a commitment. In spite of what some may claim, not all lawyers have the necessary knowledge and insight into this specialized area of a law practice.

The initial offer may be open to negotiation if the conditions appear disadvantageous to the new doctor. On the other hand, without a performance record, no starting physician should expect the same conditions, such as partnership, as the senior members of the group. However, hiring personnel do pay attention to prior research/academic records and graduation from a prestigious medical school in many cases.

8) Although a few well-regarded physicians are able to carry on their practices on a payment-at-the-time-of-service basis, most patients now have *health insurance* which covers a large part of the cost of medical care. This coverage may be provided by the patient's employer or may have been secured individually, the latter being the case especially with self-employed or unemployed persons.

To receive direct payment from the covering insurance company, the practitioner must apply for participation with the company. If accepted (which is typically the case for qualified doctors with no blemishes on their prior records), the physician will sign a contract with the insurance company. This will allow him to directly submit service *claims* to and receive payments from the insurance company. (Ways to submit claims will be discussed later.)

Applications for such participation should be submitted before beginning a practice, if possible, since there is typically a few-month-delay between application by the doctor and acceptance of participation by the company. This sort of arrangement is typical with Medicare (the national insurance plan for individuals over 65 or the disabled), Medicaid (state plans for impoverished patients), Blue Cross Blue Shield, and the majority of health insurance companies (especially health maintenance organizations – HMOs) in the market. Each requires a separate application and each will specify in what format the service claims are to be submitted. The amount of payments to be made is published according to type of service provided.

In past years, patients usually sought out particular doctors for general medical care by reputation, and the relationship continued on the strength of the doctor-patient bond. Recently, it has become more common for patients to select their doctors according to who is on their health insurance company lists.

9) In addition to malpractice insurance (which will be discussed in another chapter), **admitting privileges** at a local hospital should be sought expeditiously. This requires a formal application submission and an agreement to follow institutional regulations. An exception to acquiring such a privilege oneself is if arrangements are made for some other qualified physician to provide in-hospital care for the doctor's patients. The insurance plans in which you participate require one or the other.

10) **Equipment** needed to carry on a medical practice can be purchased outright, leased, or shared with another practitioner using the same office but on alternate days. It is sometimes possible to acquire used equipment and exam tables in good condition, especially from retiring doctors in one's geographic area. It may be necessary to take a short-term loan to cover initial expenses for startup equipment and supplies.

11) Once a practice is established, each physician will want to seek out another qualified doctor who can *cover* his practice when he is unavailable or on vacation. (Keep in mind that, by vicarious liability, the primary doctor may be held partially responsible for the covering doctor's errors made with his patients – be judicious in selecting.) If the primary doctor is also actively involved with the care of the patient at some related point, one can apportion the overall billing to the documented part each doctor actually provided. Otherwise, both may be cited for fee-splitting, which is a serious offense; Avoid calculating payments to the covering doctor as a percent of the total final charge to the patient, especially if either was not directly involved in the treatment. There is no such thing as a "referral fee" in medical practice. Alternatively, let the covering doctor bill and collect separately for the whole service he provided.

12) It is necessary for a means to be established whereby patients can reach the doctor in the case of emergency or make appointments and

receive lab results. For the former, physicians usually employ a 24/7 answering service and they carry a pager or cell phone. Appointments can either be made by the answering service or the patients can be directed to call the office at specific times when a scheduling clerk is available. Some offices work on a walk-in basis, first-come first-served.

If patients fail to keep appointments, they should be contacted for rescheduling.

13) Continuity of care: Once a physician begins treating an individual who seeks him out, a doctor-patient relationship has been established. The provider cannot avoid treating that patient in the future, even if the latter fails to pay bills, until a discontinuation of services is arranged and the patient does not object. This requires a formal notification in writing that services will be available on an emergent basis until other arrangements are made by the patient. Otherwise, the physician will be accused of *abandonment*.

14) For office employees (assistants, clerical staff, maintenance) the practice needs to carry disability, worker's compensation, and unemployment insurance. This is readily obtained through agencies of the state government in most cases and is essential coverage. Fulltime staff may need to be included in the office's health and pension plans if paid for by the practice.

15) To become known in the professional community as an up-to-date doctor, it is advisable to join the county medical society and to attend their meetings. Professional business cards should be prepared for distribution. Also, volunteering to work or lecture in a local health fair or school can help make one known in the general community.

16) Medical innovation never ceases. Thus, it is mandatory that the practicing physician continue reading professional journals which report developments in his area of medicine. Also, attending Grand Rounds at his admitting hospital will help him integrate into the professional community and maintain

knowledge of new approaches which may be incorporated into his medical practice. In some localities, participation in continuing medical education (*CME*) courses is required.

It is helpful to publicize the start of a new practice by sending formal announcements to physicians already located in the neighborhood you select. Also, local newspapers may agree to write an article about it in their publications.

It is permissible for a doctor to advertise his services. Currently, this is done with Yellow Pages® displays, direct mail brochures, and detailed websites. These modalities may enumerate the doctor's training, insurance plans, hospital affiliations, specialty, awards, office hours and locations, and publications. Ads should not be misleading, deceptive, or lacking in pertinent information.

17) A doctor must <u>never</u> claim that he guarantees a particular result (e.g., cure) from his treatment of a specific condition. Also, he should not claim expertise in any area of medicine for

which he has not received training and/or certification.

18) In addition to the HIPAA regulations (see Chap.3) which guard confidentiality of patient information, operation of a medical practice is regulated Federally by, among others:

   a) The False Claims Act;
   b) The Antikickback Statute;
   c) Stark I/II – prohibition of patient referral to other family-owned medical facilities;
   d) OSHA – medical office work safety standards;
   e) Americans with Disabilities Act; and
   f) Clinical Lab Improvement Amendments.

19) Lastly, doctors <u>must</u> avoid the personal consumption of "recreational" drugs and excess alcohol anytime during their careers since it will damage general professional reputations and may lead to sanctions by a state licensing authority. States have surveillance committees who review cases of apparent departure from acceptable physician conduct. (In New York it is called OPMC – the Office of Professional Medical

Conduct.) They have authority to impose penalties as severe as suspension of a license to practice. If a patient is harmed while the doctor is under the influence of mind-altering chemicals, he can be tried criminally.

PRÉCIS

Documents & Decisions to start a practice

1) Specialty choice
2) Group versus solo
3) Location
4) Personal liability, disability, & health insurance
5) Medical license/DEA/NPI/Social Security/EIN
6) Professional & office liability insurance
7) Health insurance company affiliation
8) Hospital admitting privileges
9) Employee disability & unemployment insurance
10) Legal rules and regulations
11) Savings/pension program

Chapter 3 – Office Record Management

Most physicians enter the practice of medicine for philosophically satisfying reasons; however, such a practice must be organized as a business to succeed and continue to provide services to the community. The proper, efficient organization and management of a medical office are essential from day #1. If the administrative side of a practice is orderly and is carried out with good business procedures, the results will benefit the doctor *and* his patients.

Several types of business data collection and keeping are necessary for personal and legal reasons. In some cases, detailed records may be needed to defend a claim or position in a malpractice suit. In other situations, the Internal Revenue Service may require the production of specific records to support items reported in tax returns.

As a doctor will hear many times in his career, an important characteristic to incorporate into his mode of practice is

DOCUMENTATION.

Although medical practice is time-consuming and compressed, the practitioner may one day thank his work style which includes detailed notes and records. The usual maxim is "if it isn't written, it didn't happen."

<u>Appointment book</u>

The first record-keeping modality is the appointment book. Because of governmental regulations (HIPAA, in particular), any medical data about a patient may not be revealed to others as verbal or written information, which includes the appointment book, without the patient's permission. (An exception to this is a formal Court order.) The appointment book is an official record of professional activities and must be kept at least as long as the Statute of Limitations is in effect. One day the doctor may be asked to display this book to prove whether a patient was seen by him or not on a particular date.

Accounting

Following an office or hospital visit, the patient will be billed for services rendered. A record must be kept of the charge, with a follow-up notation when the bill is paid.

Example: Patient Day Sheet

1/14/2008-4/14/2008

#	Date	Document	POS	Description	Provider	Code	Amount
Patient: Mary Jones							
58224	1/19/08	071219	11		1	99212	60.00
58224	1/19/08	071219	11		1	J1055	25.00
59552	3/10/08	080319		Oxford	1	03	-39.00
59553	3/10/08	080319		Adjustment	1	04	-46.00

Patient's Charges	Patient's Receipts	Adjustments	Patient's balance
85.00	-39.00	-46.00	0.00

Insurance co-pays and deductibles will typically be paid by the patient. Many offices have an explicit policy sign indicating that payment is due at the time of service. Overdue payments are typically billed by mail to the patient monthly by the doctor's office. If a charge is legitimate, it should not be written off because of billing inconvenience or inefficiency.

Delinquent patient accounts unpaid for three billing cycles should then be forwarded to a collection agency. Such firms usually have a low success rate and are limited legally to how and how much they may pressure the debtor. The doctor needs to stipulate to the collection agency that they must work within the limits of the law on his accounts. Large charges which remain uncollected after all normal attempts prove unsuccessful should result in legal action through the Small Claims Court or an attorney.

In many cases, insurance claims will be submitted on the patient's behalf, with payment being received at some later date. This is particularly true when the doctor has agreed to accept "assignment" (i.e., accept as full payment) to whatever coverage the insured may have currently. Subsequent payments can then be followed with a computer program which categorizes and times such amounts. In this way, a detailed record is kept of each transaction and, in many cases, the delinquent claims can be managed via the Internet with the insurance companies.

Some companies now insist that claims be filed online instead of on paper, and their payment is conveyed directly to the practice's business account with the bank. Where paper claims are allowed, they are usually submitted using the standardized single-page form, HCFA-1500, which is available from most medical stationery suppliers. Whether done by computer or paper, the claim must include applicable ICD and CPT codes to expedite review and payment. The wrong code may delay disbursement or result in an incorrect amount of payment:

ICD (International Classification of Disease) –

diagnosis subject codes

Sample ICD codes

V57.3 - speech-language therapy

050.9 - smallpox

733.0 - osteoporosis

757.0 - hereditary edema of legs

779.81- neonatal bradycardia

CPT (Current Procedural Terminology) –

procedure, service, and supply codes.

Sample CPT codes:

12002 – laceration suture

45355 – colonoscopy

59409 – vaginal delivery only

77051 – diagnostic mammography

99214 – extensive physical exam

These codes are commercially available in book form and are periodically revised. To get the correct payment expeditiously, one needs to use the valid, up-to-date codes. Some doctors hire commercial billing services to handle claim submission.

Many practices use a "Superbill" form which enumerates, among other items, the various possible appropriate CPT and ICD codes that could be applied for a visit or service. The form is filled out by the provider at completion of each visit and is forwarded for claim submission by the billing clerk of the office staff using this information.

Each insurance company has published allowable amounts for each procedure. This is what they will pay for a particular service by contract with the provider, regardless of the amount billed. In addition, patients are responsible for preset co-pays, deductibles, and coinsurance. The rundown of these sums is typically itemized in an EOB – Explanation of Benefits – supplied at the time of payment by the insurance company. For example, Medicare pays 80% of the allowable fee and the remaining 20% is due from the patient. (If no effort is made by the healthcare provider to collect the co-pay, Medicare argues that the *total* allowable fee should really have been 80% of the *original* allowable fee – for example, $80 instead of the original $100 allowed for a particular service, whereby the provider is really entitled to only $64 from Medicare.)

This is the ideal – but is not always realized. Insurance companies often assert that some submissions were not received by them (even if simultaneously submitted bundled with other claims that were subsequently paid) or that they are repeats of previously denied/paid claims. The medical office must rebut this if its computerized records are accurate.

A more common occurrence is the delayed payment of a charge by the patient (if not insured) or the insurance company. Typically, up to 60 days are allowed for such payment to be received following the date of claim submission. Computer programs designed for this purpose have the capacity to generate an "aging" function. (See hypothetical example below.) Once a month, the **aging schedule** is generated to show which charges are more than 60 days old. This would be followed by rebilling. If this is not done, unpaid claims can die of old age without your knowing it.

The older an unpaid charge, especially a co-pay, the less likely it will be ultimately paid. The most successful is payment of the patient's portion at the time of service.

Example: Primary Insurance Aging

As of 5/4/2010

Patient: Mary Jones   Initial billing date: 3/3/2010
SS: 101xxxxxx

Insurance: Blue Cross Blue Shield   Policy: 223xxxxxx

Date of service	Procedure	0-30	31-60	61-90	91-120	>120	Total
2/3/2010	99203	0	0	95.00	0	0	95.00

Patient: Billy Smith   Initial billing date: 3/15/210
SS: 225xxxxxx

Insurance: Oxford   Policy: AB77xxxxx

| 3/1/2010 | 99212 | 0 | 0 | 45.00 | 0 | 0 | 45.00 |

A   second   computer   program   records   **receipts,
deposits, and withdrawals** to and from your practice
account with the bank.   The total amount of each deposit
must correspond to the sum of all amounts collected on a
particular day.   Included in this program is a recording of
all outlays to cover accounts payable. Such a program

Check Register

MD PC
5/2/2011

Page 1

Date	Num	Transaction	Payment	C	Deposit	Balance
4/26/2011		Online Payment 1075600518 To Sta memo: TE FARM INS(17) cat: Insurance	290.28	R		393.47
4/27/2011		Grphealth Claimspmt 0000 memo: 10368 CCD ID: 2261330097 cat: Gr Sales		R	50.00	443.47
4/27/2011		Ghi MED/SURG Payment 0089 memo: 6097 CCD ID: 1135511997 cat: Gr Sales		R	80.00	523.47
4/27/2011		Ghi MED/SURG Payment 0089 memo: 6805 CCD ID: 1135511997 cat: Gr Sales		R	231.00	754.47
4/28/2011		Online Payment 1066105076 To memo: MOTOR FINANCE COMPANY cat: Loan Repayment	416.78	R		337.69

----

should reconcile the office account with the bank's records to be sure all posted transactions are correct.

Each physician group should have a global account for company activities, classified by provider. Also, each member of the group should have his/her own account for personal financial activities separate and apart from company functions. The two types of accounts should never be combined together, even if the practitioner is solo. To avoid mix-ups and false impressions to the IRS, these transactions must be kept separate.

Most businesses record their transactions on an *accrual* basis – expenses as they are incurred and income as it is earned. In contradistinction, medical practices typically keep their records on a *cash* basis – expenses when they are paid and income when it is actually received.

PAYROLL

Employee #	State (1-51): Local (0-6):
Name:	E/C – No, Single, Married
Street:	SDI/SUI tax (Y/N)
City/State/Zip:	Federal exempt (Y/N)
Phone:	State exempt (Y/N)
Social Soc.#:	Deduction #1:
Starting date:	Deduction #2:
Marital status (S/M/D)	Tax deferred:
Payperiod (D//W/M)	Exemptions: Fed.__ State__
Pay type (H/S)	Additional:

Computer programs are also available for employee records and payroll (see example above). Some doctors, especially in groups, use commercial firms to calculate and coordinate payrolls.

Medical Records

At the first visit, it is common procedure to have the new patient complete three sets of information which become a permanent part of the chart:

1) Insurance specifics and home address

2) HIPAA disclosure (which the patient signs)

3) Medical history (with a list of medications currently being taken – including "natural" and OTC drugs).

The data a healthcare provider collects about his/her patients in written or computerized form (including lab results) must be stored in a cabinet which is locked when the office is closed. This includes notations made from privileged verbal information. Patient privacy is insisted upon by law. In addition, new lab results must be reviewed by the practitioner (not a medical assistant) and signed soon after receipt, with a plan of action inaugurated in a timely fashion where needed.

Although it requires a significant initial investment, medical records in computerized form greatly aid data recall and reduce the loss of prior records. By 2009, 48% of office-based physicians were using EMR systems totally or in part. Several **Electronic Medical Record** (EMR) programs are now available for this purpose. They often include prescription writing and appointment listing. This approach is easiest to implement if started from the beginning of a practice.

It is important to show a continuity of care with your ongoing patients. In addition to the appointment book, a method must be instituted whereby patients are recalled by mail or phone when repeat visits are indicated (e.g., annual exams). Email may be less desirable because of the possibility of intercepted messages. If such announcements are returned to the office because of incorrect addresses, the notices should be stored in the patient's chart. If it is necessary to recall a patient because of an abnormal test result and the phone number of the client in your records is not correct or current, a registered/return receipt letter must be sent to the patient with such an alert.

Except in life-threatening emergencies, it is a standard of care to explain fully to competent patients a proposed surgical, therapeutic, or diagnostic course of action. This should be detailed on a written, witnessed, and dated **informed consent** document, and should include:

1. a statement that consent is voluntary - no penalty or denial of services if refused;

2. description of the procedure in wording or language understood by the patient;

3. purpose of the proposed procedure;

4. foreseeable risks, side effects, or discomfort;

5. expected benefit;

6. alternatives – including no procedure; and

7. confirmation that all patient questions were answered.

As with other documents, this consent becomes an official, permanent part of the patient's chart.

CHAPTER 4 – INFLATION AND COMPOUNDING –

THE *RAISON D'ÊTRE* FOR EARLY FINANCIAL PLANNING

Investments are not just for the very rich. The purpose of an investment program is not only for each person to have a place to park his/her money safely when not being used currently, but also to keep ahead of inflation. An economy expands in proportion to the productivity of its members, the flow of currency, and the internal/external demand for its products (supply versus demand). The prosperity of a country depends on the turnover (circulation) of money for the purchase of goods or services, as well as appropriate amounts of savings/investment to provide loan capital/credit for commercial expansion.

As economies prosper, so do the expectations of the workers rise within that framework. Employees are motivated by the prospect of sharing in the success of the companies in which they work so as to increase their purchasing power for desired goods and services. There is an upward pressure on salaries to meet this expectation. As a result, wages and the prices of services/goods produced often increase in parallel.

A rise in prices accompanied by a growth in the volume of money and is called "*inflation*." Barring a collapse of the overall economy or Government imposition of artificial price controls, costs always increase in the long-term. Without job promotion, salary raises, or expansion of opportunity, the initiative and the purchasing power of the employee remain static or decrease. What was obtainable previously remains the same – only the number of current dollars needed to purchase the same goods or services changes.

Although it happens much less commonly, a sharp decrease in demand can lead to *deflation* in prices.

CONSUMER PRICE INDEX (CPI)

1967 - 100

2000 - 516

2005 - 585

2010 - 653

The above table demonstrates the essence of why suitable investments are necessary – to keep even with or ahead of inflation, and the decreasing purchasing power (devaluation) of each unit of money with time (e.g., dollar, pound, euro). A convenient measure of the changing value of the currency in the United States is the Federal Government's Consumer Price Index (CPI). For example, using 1967 as the base year in which a hypothetical group of items cost $100, one can calculate what the same (or comparable) items would cost today. As noted in the table above, such an assemblage of items would cost $653 in 2010. In other words, the value of each dollar in 2010 was about 15% of what it was in 1967. Similarly, you would need 6½ times as many dollars in 2010 as you did in 1967 to purchase the same goods and services. Comparing $653 (in 2010) with $100 (in 1967) is not an increase in wealth since the purchasing power of the two at the times indicated is the same.

Rates of inflation vary from country to country. The value of a particular currency in relation to other world currencies determines the **exchange rate** between countries. Although the exchange rate is the result of several complex interacting factors, an easy way to visualize this is with the *Big Mac Index*, devised by the British publication, "The Economist." The fast food chain McDonalds® has outlets in more than 100 countries. The composition of the Big Mac® hamburger is essentially the same in all localities, but the cost of the components and of labor varies significantly; thus, if one compares the price of a Big Mac from one country to another, such a comparison must take into account most or all the factors which make up the economic variables affecting the inflation rate in the countries considered. Since this index is an attempt to measure purchasing power parity, an exchange rate higher or lower than one calculated by this method would roughly indicate if a particular currency is over- or undervalued relative to the US dollar. Similarly, it is apparent that economies are not equal worldwide.

This index can also be used to compare how long an average employee must work in each given country to buy a Big Mac.

The average inflation rate in 1980 was an unusually high 13.6%. In contradistinction, the annualized rate in the

US as of 1/2011 was 1.6%, which is relatively low historically. So as not to fall behind with money put in savings at the beginning of 2011, the vehicle for investment at that time must yield 1.6% or more per year. The short-term interest rates now (2011) offered by savings institutions are around 1% per annum or less. Other than providing safe-keeping for personal funds, one would lose monetary value trying to be secure by this means alone.

In part, this variability is one of the reasons why an investment program must be diversified with several modalities incorporated together for enhancement of one's net worth, besides accumulation of current practice income. The dominant reason for **diversification** of assets is to cushion the effects of one sector of the economy sliding while others are advancing. In addition, components of particular investment plans are not forever and need to be adjusted periodically as conditions change.

Another measure of the strength of American money is the *Dollar Index*. This parameter is the relative value of the dollar compared to six other major foreign currencies. Setting the value of the dollar in 1973 as 100, the Dollar

Index now (2011) is 74.9, showing the decrease in its value relative to the overall world economy. While today the dollar is still the preeminent standard in world trade, an increasing national debt and an enlarging international trade imbalance undermine its dependability. As a result, goods imported into the US have become relatively more expensive and American exports become more competitive in foreign markets with time. A weaker dollar should bring down the trade deficit. However, for now the US trade shortfall continues to increase because of persistently elevated borrowing.

INVESTMENT RETURN

Example: $10,000 at 4% (net)

yearend	compound	increment
1	10,400	400
2	10,816	416
3	11,249	433
10	14,800	4800
20	21,911	7111
30	32,434	10523

Let us assume one has $10,000 to put away in savings and can be guaranteed a 4% return on the total _accumulated_ balance each year for the next 30 years. (Any taxes due will be disregarded in this example.) At the end of the 1st year, investment will have earned $400 interest, for a total of $10,400.

The balance at the end of the 2nd year will be $10,816, since 4% of $10,400 (not $10,000) is $416 (i.e., $10,400 plus $416 of new interest = $10,816).

During the 3rd year it will earn $433 in interest, which is 4% of $10,816, for a yearend total of $11,249.

This is the magic of **compounding**. The more years one keeps this investment (principle + accrued interest) intact in the savings account, the more he earns in interest each successive year, compared to the previous years.

From the sample investment table above, one can readily see that the interest earned in the 2nd 10-year period ($7111) is much more than in the 1st 10-year period ($4800). By the end of the 30th year, assuming no withdrawals of principle (the original $10,000) or the accumulated interest, the total value of the account would be $32,434, more than triple the amount originally invested. On the other hand, if the investor received no interest at all, the purchasing power of the $10,000 remaining after 30 years would be much less than what it was at the beginning. In most cases, this should keep the purchasing power even with or ahead of inflation.

Investment Summary:

$10,000 for 30 years at 4% per annum

Interest type	Total accumulation
None	$10,000
Simple	$22,000
Compound	$32,434

Another example can be used to demonstrate the "Rule of 72": Assume a sum of $100 is invested at 12% interest per year. With *compounding*, the total asset would double in value (to $200) in 6 years

(72/12=6), whereas with *simple* interest it would be worth only $<u>172</u> at that time.

The take-home lessons from these examples, which could apply to any stable investment which yield interest or dividends, are:

1) Do not withdraw any increase in value (e.g., interest, capital gains, dividend) of the investment until the preplanned maturity date is reached, unless a better opportunity or emergent need arises in the interim. All gains should be <u>reinvested</u> as soon as issued. (Some assets allow automatic purchase of new units with accrued returns – hence, compounding.)

2) The earlier one begins a savings program, the larger will be the end result. The <u>rate</u> of gain increases with time (e.g., compound interest).

3) The <u>younger</u> the individual is when starting a savings/investment program, the more time there is available to make up for any unexpected mistakes or downturns that occur in

the program. A 50-year-old has less time to regain funds for retirement than a 30-year-old.

4) The initiation of a savings/investment/pension program must coincide with the startup of a medical practice, at the latest. This process is not a voluntary luxury, but is a *necessity* for future quality of life.

Chapter 5 – Investment and Savings Possibilities

TYPES

1. Mattress

2. Bank savings account

3. Money market account

4. Certificate of deposit

5. US treasurys

6. Municipal bonds

7. Corporate bonds

8. Preferred stock

9. Common stock

10. Mutual funds/ETF

11. Real estate

Various means for retaining money for future use are listed above in order of increasing rates of return on the initial investment. In addition, going down the list in general parallels an increasing relative risk of your investment (i.e., the chance of losing the principle and/or accumulated gains).

As seen recently in America, the value of real estate can vary widely and unexpectedly, sometimes profitably and at other times disastrously. On the other hand, investment in US Government securities is about the safest of all modalities in today's market because of the general strength of the American economy as well as the Government's ability to tax and borrow if needed; however, because of this low risk, the rate of potential return is lower than a well-regarded stock. (With future changes in the investment market, these generalizations may also change.)

In the United States, previously issued stocks and bonds are traded on several exchanges, depending on the size of each company and the nature of their business. The shares of more than 3000 large companies are bought and sold on the New York Stock Exchange (NYSE) and typically account for about 60% of all shares traded on the national exchanges. Securities of small-to-medium-sized companies are handled on the American Stock Exchange (AMEX). The shares of small companies not listed on an organized exchange are traded by phone and computer between brokers' offices and are monitored by the National Association of Securities Dealers (NASDAC).

The intermediaries and sources of information one should utilize to effect these transactions are covered in Chap.7.

Types of savings modalities:

1) Mattress – For accessibility, one's mattress is handy; however, security is compromised in a fire or robbery. No interest accumulates, whereby the value of the money stored this way decreases in purchasing power as inflation proceeds.

2) Bank savings account – Generally, the interest allowed is less than the inflation rate. In that the deposits are usually insured by the FDIC (Federal Deposit Insurance Corporation) up to a defined limit, the funds are secure even if a particular savings institution goes bankrupt. The cost for the insurance is typically passed on to the investor in the form of reduced returns.

3) Money market accounts – These are open-ended mutual funds (see below) which invest in short-term, highly liquid (easily cashed), reasonably safe securities. Shares in the fund can be redeemed at any time via check writing privileges. Yields are

relatively low but are usually more than in a bank savings account. Funds are not Federally insured.

4) Certificate of deposit (CD) – By law, banks must hold a specific amount of money in reserve to be able to make loans. Other than customer deposits and borrowing from the Federal Reserve, banks may obtain this money by having customers loan it to them in the form of CDs for a specified period of time at a fixed rate of interest. Bank CDs are usually Federally insured. There are penalties for withdrawal prior to term. Interest, which is typically given at a higher rate than a bank savings account but lower than bonds (see below), is taxable.

[Everyone should endeavor to have available an emergency sum for urgent, unforeseen needs (e.g., illness), generally equal to about 3-6 months of typical expenditures. These amounts can be kept in savings, money market, CD, or checking accounts for immediate use, if needed.]

5) US treasurys – On a regular basis, the US Government borrows money from various sources as bonds, if tax receipts are insufficient to cover

general expenditures. The rate of interest increases in proportion to the length of the security's term (the longer the term, the higher the rate). Such securities may be offered from as short as 3 months to more than 10 years (bills: 91-182 days; notes: 1-10 years; bonds: >10 years). Interest is exempt from state and local tax. Although selling bonds to finance spending deficits has been the primary method employed, the Federal Government also has the option of printing additional money, but this dilutes the buying power of currency already in circulation and may promote inflation.

6) Municipal bonds - Alternatively, state and local governments may issue such bonds (called municipals or "munis") for themselves, which are exempt from federal, state, _and_ local taxes if issued by the state/city in which the purchaser resides; hence, for example, a $1.00 return on a tax-free municipal bond investment would have to be $1.39 with a taxable security (assuming a Federal marginal tax rate of 28% - see Chap.6) to also net $1.00 after taxes. In other words, the amount invested in a tax-free muni needs to be much less

than a taxable bond to yield the same after-tax net return, assuming similar rates of interest. Munis are especially advantageous to investors in high income brackets, but should not be part of a deferred taxation plan (see Chap.6). If state and local taxes are included, the benefit of the tax exemption is even larger.

Most bonds (including "industrials" – see below) are rated for their relative safety by Moody's or Standard&Poor's (independent agencies) against the risk of issuer default. Unless one can tolerate the possibility of losing a portion of his savings, no bond should be purchased with a rating less than AA. Top-rated bonds (AAA) often have supplementary insurance coverage, thereby adding a measure of security.

The riskier the bond, the higher is its rate of return. However, the cautious investor should avoid purchasing speculative-grade (rated BB or lower), high-yield "junk" bonds because of their increased risk of default. Like most bonds, these securities can be sold on the open market before maturity for whatever may be the going rate.

7) Corporate bonds – To build new facilities or to aid in the marketing of existing products (especially new ones), companies often borrow money from various sources. Other than banks, the most common source of capital is the investing public. These loans are defined as bonds which are generally issued in multiples of $1000 at specific rates of return, for specific periods. Based on prevailing interest rates, such bonds may gain or lose value if sold on the open market before term. At certain preset points in the life of the bond the issuing company has the option to buy it back (call) at a defined price. A variation of this is a zero-coupon bond, which is sold initially at discount and pays interest to the holder only at the end of the term instead of periodically.

8) Preferred stock – This modality has characteristics in common with bonds (see above) and common stock (see below). They are issued by companies, especially utilities, for the same reason as bonds. Dividends are paid at a fixed rate by the company to the holder of the stock. Preferred stock, once issued, is traded in the equities market at a price

determined by its attractiveness to the investors. Principle is never repaid by the issuer but may be bought back by the issuing company at a later date (thereby eliminating dividend payout). Yield is often higher than with bonds. One significant downside to corporate dividends is that they are based on cash which is taxable both to the issuer and the recipient.

9) Common stock – These investment vehicles are issued by companies from time to time to finance a new undertaking or expand existing facilities to increase profitability. Holders of the stock vote on certain matters related to the management of the company.

Once issued, common stocks are broadly traded in various markets around the world. Prices of such shares usually vary much more widely than preferred stocks or bonds from the same companies. Over time, share prices generally attain greater appreciation than other forms of investment. If the company is very profitable and there is no immediate need for added investment in product development or production facilities by the company, dividends (profits shared with stockholders) may be larger than with preferred stock.

Trends in the price of a particular stock normally follow the anticipated progress and profitability of the underlying company; however, the psychological factor (especially fear) related to unexpected changes (such as lower-than-expected quarterly earnings) can alter this trend markedly.

New or rapidly growing companies characteristically use current profits for reinvestment in their operations rather than issuance of dividends to the shareholders. Alternatively, in the event of bankruptcy, any remaining assets are distributed first to holders of bonds, then preferred stocks, and finally, if any is left, common stock.

Over time, the value of the dollar decreases because of inflation (see Chap.4). Thus, in the long run, the overall Stock Market Average will typically rise (see graph below of Dow Jones Industrial Average of 30 large companies) in part due to this monetary depreciation.

DOW JONES INDUSTRIAL AVERAGE (1990-2011)

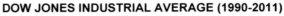

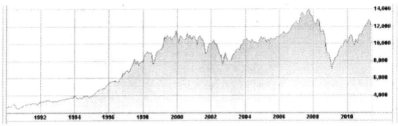

In a potentially volatile market, a "stop loss" order can be left with the brokerage firm to automatically sell a particular stock if its price falls to or below the target value selected. If a particular stock is currently at $40 per share, the holder may select a target price of $36, for example. The trade would not be executed until the price of the stock reaches $36 or less. This avoids having to incur a much larger loss if a precipitous fall occurs in a short period of time and the investor is not watching the market at that particular moment.

(Stock options ["derivatives"] are not discussed here because they are not allowed in qualified pension plans.)

Stocks can be classified by their potential for long-term, above-average growth of principle versus current income from dividends. Certain types of investments are classically known for *growth* (e.g., stock of growing companies with low/no dividends) versus *income* (e.g., high-dividend preferred stock of utilities). The balance between these two types in a particular investment programs is determined by an investor's current needs versus future anticipated requirements.

Since the potential growth in value of stocks *and* their inherent risk of loss are typically greater than bonds, a young investor would usually favor them in his portfolio. As he gets older, the balance would shift to fixed income securities such as bonds since they tend to change in open market value more gradually. The time until retirement would determine how much risk a particular investor would be recommended to undertake.

10) Mutual funds – a combined pool of money from individual shareholders for investing in a large portfolio of stocks and/or bonds of a defined type (e.g., companies dealing with energy products) which is managed by experienced brokers for the fund for a fee. Such funds offer diversification (hence, dilution of risk) since a variety of securities make up the portfolio. Shares of the fund itself are marketable or redeemable

at the end of each trading day, and gains are taxable to the participating investors (except for certain municipal bond funds). A variation of this is the ETF (Exchange Traded Funds) where fund shares can be exchanged like other securities while the Stock Market is still open during the day.

Another popular type is an Index Fund whose value passively tracks changes in a specific assemblage of securities (e.g., Dow Jones 30 Industrials) in roughly the same proportion as the group.

For the new, inexperienced investor, mutual funds are a reasonable first step in developing an investment program. They offer diversification rather than concentration in a few securities and they utilize the expertise of experienced brokers. With time, the investor himself will accumulate both net worth and knowhow, making self-management of his assets a desirable direction in which to move, for the reasons given earlier.

Dollar Cost Averaging is an investment method whereby a fixed amount of dollars is set aside at particular intervals (e.g., monthly, quarterly) in a well-managed fund with a good track record. In this way, more shares are bought automatically when the price is low and fewer when it is high.

11) Real estate – One's personal home should never be considered an investment for retirement funding since values may rise or fall before that time. Also, the individual may elect to remain in the same home without selling it after retirement. An existing mortgage should be repaid as early as possible since the interest is usually significantly higher than the inflation rate. Borrowing against the accrued value of one's house (a home equity loan) has risk of foreclosure, especially if unanticipated loan repayment problems arise at a later date. The interest on home mortgages and home equity loans remains one of the few tax-deductible items in this category.

Other desirable properties (rentable homes or apartments) can be selected for current income potential and long-term capital appreciation (increased value). The costs of purchase, mortgage payments, and maintenance can have tax advantages. On the downside, income is lost but overhead outlays continue during periods of vacancy. Timely collection of rents and eviction of nonpaying tenants are sometimes problematic.

An alternative is to invest in a publicly traded REIT (real estate investment trust). This is a professionally managed portfolio of various properties such as shopping malls and office buildings, yielding rental receipts, mortgage income, and capital gains from sales.

CHAPTER 6 – QUALIFIED PENSION PLANS AND DEFERRED TAXATION

The primary purpose of pension plans is to set aside funds during periods of active employment for later use upon retirement or prolonged disability. Current contributions to funds qualified by Government criteria are usually deductible from gross income. Investment income and capital gains taxes are deferred until withdrawal, which is one of the most important aspects of such an action.

The US tax system is graduated, meaning that the rate of taxation increases as the amount being taxed increases. The highest level (tax on the last dollar earned in a year) is the "marginal" rate (see sample table below). It is reasonable to assume in most cases that annual taxable income is less after retirement (e.g., withdrawals from a pension) than before (e.g., salary); thus, income tax on the gross investment and the accrued gains from a qualified pension investment are deferred to a much later date, when the tax rate for the individual would probably be lower.

SINGLE FEDERAL TAX RATES, 2010

Marginal tax rate	Taxable income ($)
10%	< 8,500
15%	8,500-34,500
25%	34,500-83,600
28%	83,600-174,400
33%	174,400-379,150
35%	> 379,150

The retirement plans (also called superannuation) are typically organized by and executed in banks, employer associations, insurance companies, government agencies, trade unions, investment management firms, or stock brokerage houses. (Some medical, industrial, or hospital groups administer their own programs.) Investment decisions for each plan are usually made by the investor himself, brokerage employees, or representatives of the fund.

There are currently several types of qualified pension plans that might be suitable for the practicing physician. In the first three plans (see below), the mode and rate of distribution of assets after retirement or disability may be determined by the employee. Since the accounts are established with pre-tax dollars, withdrawals are taxed at the time of distribution. An exception to this is a Roth IRA, but physicians often have earned income levels higher than the upper limit allowed by regulation to qualify for such a program.

Withdrawals before the qualifying age (usually 59½) are penalized. In some cases, funds may be withdrawn early without penalty for certain home purchases, medical expenses, college costs, and tax arrears:

1. Traditional IRA – an individual retirement savings for workers not otherwise covered by a qualified plan.

2. Keogh – a pension plan for the self-employed.

3. 401(k) – corporate employee pre-tax contributions of salary to a qualified plan, sometimes matched by the employer.

4. Social Security – a non-voluntary pension plan managed by the US Government.

5. Annuities – For the present payment of premiums, an insurance company contracts to pay the insured sums of money at a future date, which are diminished in part by processing/management fees. Like other insurance policies, premiums are determined, in part, by actuarial calculations based on the life expectancy of the insured investor. Earnings on moneys invested are accumulated tax-deferred, like other qualified plans. Future income is assured and fixed by the terms of the contract and the financial strength of the insurance company. Buying power of withdrawn money is affected by prevailing inflation rates. Such plans are most suitable for people without heirs who seek assured income for the rest of their retirement lives.

In some cases, annuities are marketed and managed by charitable organizations or universities, so that the contributions to the plan by the insured may be tax-deductible when given.

Although not strictly a pension plan, a qualified "529" tax-advantaged state savings program can be set up for the college education of dependents. Taxation is not imposed upon withdrawal if the funds accumulated in the plan are used for college expenses only. Invested money is not insured and is subject to market risks.

QUALIFIED PENSION PLANS

(deferred taxation)

1. IRA – individual retirement plan

2. Keogh – plan for the self-employed

3. 401k – corporate employee contribution plan

4. Social Security – mandatory US government plan

5. Annuity

Chapter 7 – Advisors and Brokers

In that laymen are not fully knowledgeable in all aspects of finance and the law, certain advisers should be consulted from time to time in evolving and maintaining investment activities. Selection of candidates can depend on recommendations from colleagues.

1. Stock brokers – There are basically two types of stock brokerage firms: *full service* and *discount*. In the first case, the broker and his coworkers are called upon to provide advice on specific selections of stocks and bonds to purchase or sell based on the research facilities within their company. On the other hand, discount brokers only execute trades (often via the Internet) in and out of an account based on the investor's independent decisions. The difference in fees for the same trade between the two types of brokers can be as much as 30-to-1. Such a commission range can make the

difference between net gains and losses for the same trade.

2. Certified Financial Planners – These advisers, often part of the staff of a brokerage firm, must pass a 3-step qualifying exam demonstrating their ability to counsel on financial planning, insurance, banking, investments, and taxes. The most objective CFP is usually one who charges a set *hourly* fee rather than a *commission* on execution of suggested transactions. Commissioned planners only make money if assets are bought or sold in the investor's account. It is advisable that all final decisions about trades be in the hands of the asset owner rather than the adviser or broker.

3. Lawyers knowledgeable in estate planning (see Chap.10).

4. Accountants – The doctor whose sole income is salary and whose deductions are

standard can usually process his own taxes, especially with computer programs now available. More complicated practices, because of periodic changes in the law and the complexity of business returns, need the attention of a certified public accountant (CPA).

5. Self-study – The newspaper, TV, or radio should never be solely relied upon for information to be used in making financial decisions. Once it is publicized, everyone knows about it and any insightful advantage is lost.

There are many modalities available for learning the ins-and-outs of investment. A number of websites provide virtual investment programs to help the novice become accustomed to trading securities hypothetically. Many books have been published on the approaches to managing investment accounts and personal assets.

Books that should be avoided are those that promote a get-rich-quick method for making a killing in the market. Budgeting techniques require a sensible balance between income, necessary expenditures, savings, and luxuries.

6. Advisories – The most useful sources of investment information are those that objectively present data on business history, share price, P/E ratio (price per share/earnings per share), recent dividends, financial status, product development, and manufacturing functions of many companies which have securities traded on the stock exchanges (e.g., Value Line®). Rather than promoting specific investments, such sources provide the information that the doctor can utilize to make an educated determination on his own.

Example: GENERAL ELECTRIC CO.®

as of 4/28/2011

Today's Open	$20.72
Previous Close	$20.60
Day's Range	$20.40 - $20.74
52 Week range	$13.75 - $21.65
Beta	1.65
Earnings per Share (04/21/2011)	$1.20
Price/Earnings	17.04
Quarterly Dividend (Ann. Yield)	$0.15 (2.93%)

Above is a portion of a typical example of information regularly available from stock brokerages and data suppliers. It is relatively easy to learn how to interpret these charts and use them to determine the value of each security. The independent investor should be able to use these data readily to make investment decisions on a regular basis.

7. The sound investor should not rely on "off-the-cuff" tips or hunches of his own or

of his associates and friends. Investing, if diversified into several categories of industry and finance, is not a "crap shoot" or a game of darts. The educated, informed investor much more often gains than loses in the long term.

PRÉCIS

ADVISORS/BROKERS

1. Full service vs. discount broker

2. Profession advisor – commission vs hourly

3. Virtual learning programs/books –

    Avoid get-rich-quick schemes or advisories;

    If it sounds too good to be true, it probably is.

4. *Best:* Manage your own assets with

    knowledge, not hunches or tips.

    (or give Bernie Madoff a call)

CHAPTER 8 – INVESTMENT GUIDELINES

Based on his own real-life experiences, the author has evolved an approach to personal investments. These ideas may be applicable, totally or in part, to other healthcare providers seeking to establish a workable investment approach to attaining and retaining economic stability. One size does *not* necessarily fit all.

Most individuals have little control over world events and economic changes occurring locally or internationally from day to day; however, in the long run, one has to assume that his professional activities, if managed consistently and diligently, can lead to a steady improvement of lifestyle and establishment of a secure future for himself and his dependents. The lottery is suitable for a fortunate few, but for most of us mortals, coordinated, independent effort establishes a solid foundation for comfortable living and a satisfying career.

Many years are dedicated by doctors to reach the capability of applying medical knowledge for the betterment of other human beings. So too, knowledge in the economic realm will lead to the development of a program of sustained personal growth and achievement of goals outside the profession.

From the beginning of a career, money available for personal spending should be budgeted into two groups: *essentials* and *discretionary*. The former includes food, shelter, and clothing; the latter encompasses the "fun" things like vacations and entertainment. Based on actual anticipated income, a budget should be derived which takes into account these two groups. Regular monitoring of expenditures can point to needed adjustments (see example below).

Advisors often say that investors need to set goals and objectives for their financial program. The easy answer is to say,"to make money"; however, most of life's defining events are not predictable, such as health problems, law suits, and the inflation rate. Thus, it is necessary for each person to comprehend his true (not hypothetical) **current** economic situation and project roughly certain anticipated expenses, such as feeding

Create – and stay – on budget

Track Spending Goals to Save Money

◄ July 2010 ►

		Goal	Remaining
Total	$567	$700	$133
Auto		100	100
Clothing	79	100	21
Dining	140	400	260
Entertainment	274	50	274 over
Groceries		50	26

Reproduced with permission by Quicken® (Intuit, Inc.)

one's family and covering future educational outlays.

In particular, children's tuition costs are difficult to estimate many years in advance, but some funds must be reserved for this purpose. As realities become apparent and careers progress, modifications should be made, but this is only feasible if a savings/investment program has been established *early* to allow accumulation of net worth for future needs.

Computer programs exist that help one predict how his current and projected rate of savings/investments may or may not satisfy his needs after retirement (see example above). These require the person to estimate his future monetary needs and the expected mean rate of inflation.

1) Never *accept* advice blindly; research investment decisions before execution. Avoid tips and hunches from others. Never *give* advice → how to keep friends from hating the source of costly misinformation.

2) Never become too attached to a failing security. Admit an error, pull out, and move on. Many months may pass if the investor is waiting for a depressed stock to regain its original purchase price before selling it. The money gleaned early from its sale may gain value much faster if now invested in a more productive security. No one selects correctly 100% of the time. Trades must be made as objectively and unemotionally as possible.

3) One's money should be working for him maximally 24/7 through **diversification** of assets.

4) Check the performance of asset holdings at least <u>twice a week</u>, not once a quarter. With the Internet, this is easy. Determining <u>when to sell</u> an asset, not when or what to buy, is the toughest of all investment decisions.

5) Never look back. (The Bible tells of a woman who turned to salt when she did.) Cash in hand is worth more than on paper. A gain in value is only realized when the asset is sold, not when the current value exceeds the original purchase price.

6) Learn and refine how to manage finances as diligently as a practitioner learned how to manage his patients. Investing is a tool for achieving economic security for his family as much as is his practice income. It is not a hobby.

7) *Avoid unmanageable debt.* Each practitioner should pay off student loans on time, live within his income limits, and resist easily obtained high-interest-rate credit card debt.

8) Do not be diverted from a rational investing program by "herd" mentality, such as the Internet dot-com financial bubble, which collapsed in 2001 faster than it formed.

9) The decision to invest in a particular stock could depend on the company's prospects for continued growth (e.g., new drugs) or by price trend technical analysis.

10) "Penny" stocks are high-risk securities typically priced at less than $5 per share. Although every novice investor dreams of discovering the next Microsoft® in the early stages, penny stocks, like "junk" bonds (see Chap.5), are to be avoided because of their unacceptable failure rate.

CHAPTER 9 – INSURANCE

There are several types of insurance a doctor will need to consider during his/her professional years, some of which must be in place on day #1 of practice. The main purpose of such coverage is to protect personal assets so that that the practitioner will not be made destitute because of an unfortunate event in his personal or professional life.

<u>Malpractice</u>

First among these is malpractice insurance. Most hospitals and health insurance companies will not allow a doctor to treat his patients without suitable coverage. (Some states do allow doctors to "go bare", but these are the exception.) The premium paid for such insurance is a tax-deductible practice expense. There are basically two types of policies:

Occurrence: This policy is in effect for the duration of the Statute of Limitation for initiation of a suit (the time after which a plaintiff can no longer file a suit following the event in question) if the occurrence took place while the policy was in force. Premiums are higher than claims-made (see below). Indemnity coverage remains in effect for events taking place during the coverage period even after termination of the policy. In the absence of tort reform, it is likely that premiums will continue to rise in the foreseeable future.

Claims-made: Events are covered only if the suit is filed in the incident year when the policy is active. Additional "tail" coverage is needed for suits filed later than one year. Initially, premium for the basic claims-made policy is lower than for the occurrence type, but eventually rises in the subsequent years as the tail coverage is continued.

Some malpractice insurance companies offer discounts to new physicians in their first year of medical practice and for those taking risk management courses. Also, doctors working in their practices (actual patient contact) less than 20 hours a week may be eligible for premium reductions of 25-50% in certain cases.

Potential malpractice suits are a reality of contemporary medical practice. In a study done a few years ago, it was found that 47% of all Board-certified obstetricians in New York had been sued at least *four* times during their careers. The insurance company normally covers the costs of litigation. Suit settlements and judgments, as well as disciplinary actions related to incompetence and professional misconduct, are recorded in the National Practitioners Data Bank. The information is confidential and is only available to hospitals, state licensing boards, and certain healthcare entities.

A malpractice suit may be filed if the events in question appear to bear four key characteristics:

1. A doctor-patient relationship exists, creating a *duty* to perform a service.

2. As determined by accepted standards of care, a *breach* in the performance of that duty occurs.

3. Monetary, emotional, or physical *damage* to the patient results from the breach.

4. A *proximate cause-and-effect* relationship between the performance and the damage can be identified.

According to classical Kantian ethics, the performance of a duty is more important than the results, good or bad. However, modern juries judge an adverse outcome by whether or not it conformed to "normal" standards of medical practice in the community (by whatever measure that may be defined). In addition, the subjective opinions of testifying "experts" are still held as admissible, rather than analysis exclusively grounded in evidence-based medical research. (Clearly, a more objective standard is needed.)

Health

Doctors and their family members do get sick from time to time. Although it used to be common practice for doctors to treat each other, as needed, on a "professional courtesy" basis, such reciprocity is less common now; therefore, it is important for every doctor to have an active family health insurance policy in effect at all times. For those joining groups or employed by hospitals, this benefit is commonly given as part of the association agreement. In addition to basic coverage, a "catastrophic" major medical policy should be obtained as well. The latter type of policy is inexpensive and becomes priceless should the need arise.

There are several types of coverage available. Some only pay for expenses incurred while hospitalized, whereas others cover both in-patient and out-patient care. A number do not bear the cost of well-patient checkups. Health Maintenance Organizations (HMOs) typically encourage annual exams, whereby conditions are uncovered and are usually more easily (less expensively) treated in the earliest stages.

Disability

The third type of insurance that the practitioner MUST have from the beginning of his career is disability coverage. Whereas life insurance (to be discussed below) is needed early in one's professional life (especially while still in medical training if there are dependents), disability insurance is even more important. A disabled "bread-winner" not only fails to bring home earnings, he/she must be fed for prolonged periods too, particularly if the disability is permanent.

When filling out an application for disability insurance, it is important to list as one's profession the most complicated activity he commonly does (e.g., cardiac catheterization); thus, if he is unable to do caths, the doctor would be classified physically as "disabled." He would be eligible for disability compensation, even though he may be able to work part-time at less demanding activities such as EKG readings or delivering lectures.

It is highly advisable that individuals should document in a legally defensible form his/her wishes in the event of incapacitation. Most people have preferences for who should make healthcare decisions for them (health proxy) and what their wishes are (living will) under life-threatening conditions. This should be formalized in writing *before* the need arises.

<u>Personal Liability</u>

In addition to the various insurances a doctor will need to obtain for his medical practice, he must arrange for liability coverage in the office and home setting – e.g., a slip-and-fall injury in the waiting room. An economical way to deal with this is to have an "***umbrella***" liability policy which takes over if the claims of liability exceed basic coverage in the home, office, or car. Primary liability protection is necessary for *personal* (nonprofessional) activities. A supplementary umbrella policy would thereby provide much larger coverage at a reasonable cost. (It is amazing at how many victims of minor auto accidents develop neck pain *de novo* when they find out the other driver is a doctor!) This type of insurance has no relationship to professional malpractice coverage.

Life

Life insurance (which should be called "death" insurance) is important for the family if the doctor is one of the main providers in his household. Most people just starting out in a medical career have little or no savings (i.e., no estate). If the primary provider dies at this point without dependents (e.g., wife and children), his parents will mourn for him but no one will go hungry; If he does have dependents, they may be left destitute. To avoid such an unfortunate financial consequence, life insurance provides an *instant estate* for those left behind. Death of young people by disease or accident is unusual but not impossible. (Suicide is not covered.)

There are tax advantages if the beneficiaries of the policy are made the owners of the policy as well. The premiums for healthy young people (such as most new doctors) are very low, so that coverage for at least $1M should put little strain on a budget. (Life insurance for dependent minor children is usually not necessary.)

Although they go by many different names because of slight variations between them, there are basically two types of life insurance: term and whole life. _Term_ policies provide only a death benefit. If a policy with a $1M payout is purchased, that is all the beneficiaries get, and this does not require court action (probate) which can go on for a year or two after the insured's demise. The policy has no cash value if the holder stops paying the premium while still alive.

On the other hand, _whole life_ policies have two parts:

1) a death benefit, and

2) a savings plan.

The accumulated cash value persists even if the policy is cancelled. The premium for a whole life policy is typically many times larger than a term policy because of the savings plan feature.

Generally, one could do better investing the difference between the two types of policies himself, since the premium of the whole life program includes service fees for the investment people working in the insurance company. If the insured manages his own investment affairs, he will save this avoidable expenditure. The only people who may benefit from a whole life policy are those who just cannot control themselves enough to put money away in savings on their own.

Insurance salesmen like to show potential clients how much cash value they will have in their accounts after a number of years, but a realistic calculation should be made for a term policy combined with an investment program which the insured alone manages. Similarly, for the same premium, a term policy will yield a larger death benefit for the dependents than the payout from a whole life policy (death benefit plus accrued cash value) upon one's demise. After several years in medical practice, a diligent savings plan will build up an actual estate with significant net worth, making the continuation of life insurance of any type much less necessary to protect dependents.

Early acquisition of medical and life insurance usually guarantees continued coverage at the standard premium even if a major health problem arises soon thereafter. Most life insurance policies contain a waiver of premium clause which takes effect if the insured is disabled. (The same holds true for medical malpractice and disability insurance.)

<u>PRÉCIS</u>

INSURANCE –

To protect your assets

1. Malpractice

2. Health

3. Disability

4. Personal liability

5. Life

Chapter 10 — Asset Protection/Estate Planning

In earlier chapters it was noted that half the battle is earning an income and the other half is keeping it. More so than most income-earners, doctors are targets for individuals seeking to find an excuse to usurp assets owned by the physician, by whatever means are necessary. This is commonly one of the main (unspoken) motives in malpractice claims. This is not to say that many suits are not based on legitimate reasons, since some therapeutic processes do cause unintentional untoward outcomes. Juries decide negligence. Whatever the issue, the assault on one's personal assets is possible if the damages allowed exceed the practitioner's liability insurance coverage.

As a result of this persistent threat in the background, many (probably most) doctors unfortunately practice "defensive" medicine. Marginally indicated tests, studies, and pharmaceuticals are ordered. Questionable repeat visits are scheduled. Probably more than any other factor, this environment has led to a large increase in the cost of medical care (private and public) in the United States, even though the various measures applied to evaluate the quality of healthcare in America show no significant lead (e.g., avoiding premature delivery) over other countries with less costly socialized programs.

To reduce this threat, doctors must create asset protection mechanisms *before* suits are filed to guard their future welfare from such assault. Some of these various approaches are as follows:

1) Qualified pension plans (see Chap. 6) can only be invaded by the Court in divorce proceedings or by the IRS for delinquent tax payments; otherwise, creditors are excluded.

2) An irrevocable trust is a formalized relationship where one person (the trustee) holds title to property of a donor (e.g., the parent) for the benefit of another (the beneficiary, such as one's child); thus, the property is no longer his but is held in trust until the beneficiary is qualified to deal with it, as determined by the trustee.

3) Limited liability companies (LLC) are legal entities formed (such as within families) where

each member shares assets protected from attack if the other members do not agree to a distribution. This mechanism may avoid the delays due to probate and estate taxes upon death of one of the members as well.

An estate planning expert may be consulted to ascertain the advisability of such a move. Many state governments have telephone help hotlines to guide applicants through the relatively straightforward registration process.

4) According to current American law, assets can be exchanged tax-free between legally married spouses. The property wholly in the name of the wife, for example, cannot be attacked for the liabilities of her husband. Although the continuation of a marriage can never be guaranteed, this mechanism can be useful for protecting the assets of a happily married couple which are not part of an irrevocable trust or a qualified pension plan of either member.

5) A prenuptial agreement only protects ownership of assets of one partner from the other

obtained prior to the marriage in cases where a division of property is declared in a divorce proceeding. This is especially important if the marriage comes before medical school graduation since lifetime potential income resulting from the professional degree can become an issue.

6) Schemes for hiding assets in "offshore" accounts are much less secure than they were before the US Government began obtaining information on such foreign accounts recently.

7) Industrial concerns incorporate to shield their directors from law suits against the activities of the company they direct. Whereas, professional corporations (PC) require all shareholders to be licensed in the profession, such as a group of doctors working together, they do not shield personal assets from malpractice suits against any of its members.

8) Actions which are illegal or unethical are not necessarily covered by medical malpractice insurance.

9) Recent legislation prohibits the rapid transfer of assets in anticipation of application for Medicaid coverage for a disabling or terminal condition. The gradual irrevocable transfer of assets well before the onset of care helps in qualifying for Medicaid insurance should the need arise.

10) A designation of beneficiaries can be drawn up with savings and pension accounts without a lawyer. This avoids the delays and expenses connected with probate of wills or dying intestate (without a will or other designation). As stipulated by each state's law, surviving spouses are entitled to a specific minimum of their partner's assets upon death. Charities can also be designated as tax-free beneficiaries. One of the main functions of a will is to identify who will be responsible for the care of children if no parents are surviving. (Suggestion: both parents should never fly together in the same plane if possible.)

11) Certain law firms specialize in estate planning. Since the regulations in this area tend

to be complex, consultation with such experts is advisable as one's net worth (i.e., inheritable estate) reaches significant levels.

CHAPTER 11. CLINICAL CORRELATES

The points raised in this book are best understood if illustrated with realistic situations. If this book was read carefully, the reader should be able to determine how these predicaments (indicated by *) could have been avoided or reduced, if at all. Discussions of the cases are found at the end of the scenarios. The events and characters to be described here are all fictitious; names have been changed to protect the unenlightened.

Problems

1) A 28-year-old, right-handed male is in his second year of an orthopedic surgery residency. While skateboarding in short sleeves, he fell, causing a 2x4 cm bleeding abrasion of his left elbow. Following cleaning and dressing of the wound in the ER, he was placed on oral dicloxacillin and received a tetanus vaccination. Twelve days later, the wound had not closed and was now swollen and tender. Cultures taken at the time of the original ER visit revealed MRSA, with no antibiotic sensitivity identified. (No one had taken the time to look up the culture result as yet.*) It was elected to debride

the wound. After several months of repeated treatments (once almost leading to partial reduction of the ulnar bone), the wound slowly closed and symptoms subsided. He did not regain full use of his left arm and had to change his residency to psychiatry, after being out of postgraduate training for one full year. He had health insurance to cover these treatments but had no disability coverage*. The insurance company refused to pay disability benefits.

2) A 41-year-old, unmarried, childless female obstetrician had a very successful solo practice. She had standard Obs malpractice claims-made coverage ($1M/incident; $3M/year total) with no "tail."* Her yearly practice profits were divided evenly between a mutual bond fund (not qualified as a pension plan*) and her hobby of stamp collecting*. In addition, she had an IRA account with a brokerage firm worth $10,000, rented an apartment, and had no other significant assets or savings. She delivered a baby at 26 weeks of gestation following unsuccessful tocolysis, which ended up with persistent cerebral palsy. She was

subsequently sued. Two months later, she transferred all her bond fund holdings into the IRA pension account.* After three years, a judgment for $20M was handed down against her alone in a jury trial, which was subsequently reduced to $9.5M on appeal. Her state had no fund for neurologically impaired children.

3) Dr. A.B. See, a middle-aged, married dermatologist, has placed all* his savings in a stock portfolio managed independently* by his broker at a full-service* firm. On the advice of a friend, he carefully evaluated his account for the previous year and found that 420 trades had been executed, with a net return, after expenses, commissions, and taxes, of 1.1%. Upon noting this, he became irate*, gave the order to sell all* the stock, and deposited the proceeds in a 2-year bank CD paying 1.5%. He has his attorney prepare a will* in which all his assets are left to his brother*.

4) A 29-year-old single parent completed her training in family practice and entered a group practice which initially offered her no benefits* beyond a

base salary. Her husband was a construction worker who had died in an auto accident two years previously, leaving his entire legacy of $19,500 to their daughter*. The doctor developed an especially aggressive form of ovarian sarcoma and passed away within four months. She died intestate* and her child was forced to live in a foster home at government expense since no other family members could be located.

5) Dr. R.U. Alert, an elderly psychiatrist, completed evening office hours. His support staff forgot to shut the electronic medical records computer program* before closing up the facility. Later that night, the office was burglarized and the computer containing personal information about the patients was entered. A few weeks later, one of the patients was contacted by an unknown source with a threat of blackmail.

6) A second-year medical student had read extensively on astute stock investing. After careful study, he used half of his savings from summer work to buy stock of a well-regarded, large company in the Dow

Jones Industrial 30 list. In the first three months, the stock rose 20%; however, after an unfavorable published review* by an investment guru, the stock price dropped by 3% in two days. The student sold his entire* holding, only to find the stock rise by 10% over the next 30 days.

7) A student who just completed his internship and passed his Board exams was applying for his first license to practice. On his application he conveniently neglected to mention* a prior conviction for DUI before starting medical school. In spite of an outstanding student loan of $200,000, he ran his total balance on three credit cards* to $43,000.

8) Dr. I.M. Hungry, a 56-year-old physician, had just been notified that during the 2009-2010 severe recession in the US, the value of his pension plan had decreased 20%. By an approximate projection, he believed that he will not have enough to retire at 62, as he had previously planned. His brother-in-law* told him about an investment program which promised to yield returns of 12-15% per annum*. A

quick guesstimate indicated that this program would put him back to where he was before the recession in just two years.*

9) A 43-year-old certified nurse practitioner/midwife agreed to help her client do a home delivery of her third baby. The previous births have progressed normally in a hospital setting. The patient confirmed in writing that she was aware that a home birth was riskier than a hospital-based delivery. A Board-certified obstetrician with admitting privileges at the local hospital agreed to be on call if needed when the labor ensued. The pregnancy had been uncomplicated. At 41 weeks of gestation, the patient telephoned the midwife saying that the membranes had ruptured with clear fluid observed. The nurse-midwife arrived at the patient's home in 15 minutes later to find her lying unconscious in a pool of blood. An emergency service ambulance was called. Upon arrival at the hospital, both the mother and baby were dead. Question: should the obstetrician and/or the midwife be held liable for the outcome?*

10) A young cardiologist had recently opened his solo practice near a retirement community in Florida. One of his first patients complained of increasing fatigue, lightheadedness, and dyspnea on exertion. An EKG revealed a bradyarrhythmia requiring insertion of a pacemaker. Symptoms were markedly relieved. The patient's insurance was billed for these services but it was found that the policy had been terminated prior to the treatment.* When the patient was called, he said he would make payments, but none was ever received.*

11) A Los Angeles general surgeon decided to take a 2-week vacation. He spent the first week in Canada and the second in Mexico. While in Canada, the exchange rate between the US dollar and the Canadian dollar rose by 3% in favor of the Canadian currency. While in Mexico, the foreign exchange rate between the peso and the US dollar fell by 3% in favor of the US. What investment opportunity might this present?

      a) Exchange $10,000(US) for Canadian money

b) Exchange $10,000(US) for Mexican money

c) Do neither

Discussion

Problem: 1) a) Check lab results promptly. To delay may prove to be an indefensible departure from accepted standards of medical care.

b) Disability insurance should be arranged early in a career.

2) a) By the nature of the specialty, obstetrics in many states has a Statute of Limitations of 10 years or more. If a suit is filed after the year of the event, a claims-made policy must have a "tail" or there is no coverage for the doctor. In that case, personal assets can be attacked.

b) Protection of assets from suits, such as a qualified pension plan, is essential.

c) Exposed assets are subject to attack in law suits and must be shielded with available legal methods.

d) Assets transferred into a qualified pension plan *after* the initiation of a law suit are not protected from attack by a creditor in a case with a judgment greater than the coverage limit of the insurance. Also, at age 41, the annual contribution to a Traditional IRA is limited to $5000.

3) a) Securities should be divided into more than one account for safety.

b) Management of assets must be under the ultimate control of the investor.

c) Full-service brokers have higher transaction fees (commissions) than discount brokers, but the latter offer less advice and research assistance.

d) Investment decisions need to be as objective as possible. "Spur-of-the-moment" transactions must be considered unemotionally.

e) Retention of some shares of a solid stock being liquidated may allow for later gain with less overall downside risk.

f) Beneficiary designation is best done in an official document separate from a will to avoid delays in prolonged probate. Brokerage houses have these forms available.

g) A surviving wife is typically entitled to a significant portion of her late husband's legacy even if not stipulated explicitly.

4) a) Life insurance is especially necessary early in a career when there are dependents.

b) In most situations with new graduates where there are young children, assets in a legacy should be left to a spouse to avoid possible taxation; however, with small estates, it is not likely the inheritance tax-free limits will be exceeded. An alternative would be a managed trust fund for the children.

c) A will is necessary to stipulate child custody preferences.

5) According to Federal HIPAA regulations, patient records must be guarded and locked against unauthorized intrusion in public and private areas.

6) a) To rely on so-called "experts" invites late or unreliable investment moves.

b) Usually, investment decisions should be based on trends over time, not extemporaneous hunches.

7) a) All entrees on a medical license application <u>must</u> be complete and truthful, since they become part of a doctor's permanent professional record.

b) Easily available credit card debt must be avoided because of the high interest rate.

8) a) Investment decisions need to depend on reliable sources of information. If a proposed program promises an unbelievable rate of return, it is unbelievable. Friends and relatives want to be

helpful but, in most cases, should not be the primary source of investment information for social and economic reasons.

b) Projections should be based on accurate determinations, not guesses.

9) This case demonstrates the quandary faced by qualified practitioners in today's world. While the patient was fully informed and accepted the known complications of such a proposed procedure, the emotional element especially inherent in cases involving babies often overrides objective logic. The outcome of this legal case could be very dissimilar in different parts of the country and with different juries in the same city. As a result, medical practice has become very defensive and conservative, in spite of good intentions by the practitioners. Like other emergent events in medicine, the nature of obstetrical deliveries can change very rapidly, often in ways that cannot be dealt with effectively outside a fully equipped

hospital. In most communities, the standard of care calls for such a setting to be utilized.

10) a) Diagnostic, therapeutic, and operative procedures should be precertified with the patient's insurance company to avoid nonpayment.

b) It gets progressively more difficult to collect on debts the longer the time between service and contact to effect payment. Debtor laws in most states are limiting in types of approaches that can be used. Ultimately, a lien on the debtor's credit may be the only legal recourse.

11) Next to commodities (natural resources; agricultural products) and derivatives (options to buy or sell particular stocks at fixed prices), the foreign exchange (forex) market is potentially the most capricious type of investment vehicle available. The primary purpose of the foreign exchange market is to fund international trade via banks, governments, and global companies. The daily worldwide turnover is about $4 trillion.

However, as an investment modality, forex forecasting is very difficult because past history may have little bearing on current daily changes. Marked short-term variations may hinge on destabilizing weather, politics, interest rates, inflation, or rumors. Thus, the average small investor with risk-aversion might do better with stocks and bonds.

CHAPTER 12. CONCLUSIONS:
PLAN OF ACTION FOR
THE PRACTICING DOCTOR

SUMMARY OF SUBJECTS COVERED

- PRACTICE – solo vs. group.

- MANAGEMENT – organized business procedures.

- INSURANCE – securing an instant estate.

- BUDGETING – effective control of cash flow.

- INVESTMENTS – self-directed growth of savings.

- PENSION – deferring income for future needs.

- ASSET PROTECTION – shield from potential assault.

- NET WORTH – growth of personal wealth.

- ETHICS – compassionate care.

This text has been organized to present an introduction into issues that should concern both the new and the established practitioner. It has served its objective if the reader is now at least aware of the subjects which deserve closer scrutiny and mastery to insure a life of comfort, security, and physical contentment, as a complement and aid to professional achievement. Generating, instituting, and comprehending a timetable of priorities (see abbreviated list above) _before_ the startup of an office or clinic will expedite the establishment of a rewarding practice.

In summary, the individual must be informed so that he is ultimately the master (at least in part) of his own fate.

If the reader of this book is a student doctor (medical student or resident), he is still in the formative years in terms of developing professional and personal behavior traits. The practice of medicine is a privilege whereby his patients give him the *right* to touch their bodies and their lives in a way not accessible to most other people with whom they interact. It should never be the doctor's attitude that his knowledge, expertise, and professional status entitle him to deal with his patients on anything other than an equal person-to-person plane.

Over the years in practice, the author has evolved a set of guidelines not only for managing the financial affairs of his practice, but also the personal aspects in his dealing with his patients. These ethical considerations are now directed toward **YOU**, the healthcare provider.

Random thoughts on being a good physician:

1) Be modest. In spite of the volumes you have already learned, there is much you have not as yet touched, regardless of your stage of education or experience. Your medical training and learning do not end the day you finish your residency. Due to scientific progress, the medicine I practice today has significantly advanced from what I learned during my formal training. Read, read, read.

2) Be aware that medical diagnosis is often not as clear-cut as the textbooks seem to say. In many cases, you will have

an impression based on past experience but it will lack solid scientific certainty. "Primum non nocere" – first, do no harm, i.e., practice nonmaleficence. As stated in the Hippocratic Oath: "…abstain from doing harm." It is sometimes better to do nothing than to take dubious risks. For any physician, decision-making in tenuous situations may prove to be the most difficult part of a practice.

3) Be humble. There is only one G-d in this world, and you are not He! Your patients are dependent on your expertise to keep them alive - do not take advantage of that arrangement because of your ego.

4) The basic science courses in medical school have given you a subconscious intuition into the mechanisms of disease. To diagnose the cause of an abnormal state requires a thorough understanding of the normal.

5) In some situations you will do your best for your patient and still they will not get better. Admit to your limitations; your patients will respect you for your honesty. Pay attention to the smallest details since they may hold the key to successful diagnosis and treatment.

6) Do not delude your patients if you do not know the answer to a question. Look it up before opening your mouth. Admit your mistakes. Seek consultation as needed.

7) Your medical practice will ultimately make you a millionaire. Do not squeeze your indigent patients. Try doing pro bono work once in a while, as needed.

8) The practice of medicine is unique among the professions. Society owes you *nothing* because you sweated out several years in training. You did it because you wanted the satisfaction of helping your fellowman. If that is not your motivation, try some other occupation or profession.

9) Secure your financial future by starting a savings/pension plan the day you open your practice. The big boat or luxury house can wait.

10) Patients are people, not diagnoses ("the gallbladder in room #302"). Address your patients by their surnames until they allow you otherwise.

11) Be honest in dealing with your patients and with your financial affairs. Record ALL amounts received in your

practice, including cash. You can eat only three meals a day. If you are dishonest in your financial dealings, how can your patients expect you to be honest with them in their hour of need?

12) In your role as physician and healthcare provider, your patients will often see you as superior to themselves. Avoid paternalism. This is not permission for you to take advantage of them in any form (social, physical, or economic). Make your patient a partner with you in your diagnostic process.

GLOSSARY

Accounts payable – amounts owed by the practice to other people.

Accounts receivable – amounts owed to the practice by others.

Board-certified – proven by training and examination to have met the national standards of a specialty board.

Capital gains – increase in value of an asset other than interest/dividends.

Certificate of deposit – loan to a bank at a fixed rate and term.

CPA – certified public accountant.

Commodities – natural resources, agricultural products.

Concierge – a type of health plan where a fixed amount is prepaid to a physician for unlimited care of common conditions.

Derivatives – a purchased option to buy or sell a security at a predetermined price.

Dividend – distribution of company earnings to shareholders.

Equity – value of ownership share in a corporation or an asset (e.g., stock).

Estate tax – tax paid on an inheritance by the recipient (other than assets willed to a spouse or a charity).

Fixed income – rate of interest remains the same throughout the term of the security (e.g., bonds).

Forex – foreign currency exchange market.

Gift tax – tax paid by the giver on value of anything granted to another (except spouse) in excess of a Federally fixed amount.

HCP – healthcare provider.

HIPAA – Health Insurance Portability and Accountability Act – Federal legislation to protect patient privacy and confidentiality. (In certain cases, information about teenage patients cannot be released to their parents if the children deny such access. In some states, teens may obtain medical services without parental consent, such as contraception, STD treatment, and prenatal care.)

HMO – health maintenance organization: Aside from offering comprehensive insurance coverage, these groups emphasize the role of the primary care practitioner for general treatment and for decisions regarding specialist involvement ("gate keeper").

Hospitalist – a doctor who practices exclusively as an employee of a hospital, caring for patients referred to that institution by other office-based physicians.

Inflation - A rise in prices accompanied by a growth in the volume of money and credit.

Intestate – to die without a will or formal beneficiary designation.

Liquidity – ease of converting an asset into cash.

Net worth – total value of all possessions and assets minus debts.

Probate – to establish the authenticity and intents of a will in Court.

Statute of Limitations – maximum length of time a law suit can be initiated after the event in question. For example, in New York, most medical malpractice actions must be brought within 2½ years from the date they become apparent.

Term – the preset duration of a bond or CD.

Utility – a supplier of water, gas, or electricity.

Acknowledgements: The author wishes to thank the following for their constructive reviews of this manuscript - Marvin Levine, DO, Karen Admon, RN/CNM, and Judith Binstock, PhD.

Index

QUICK ORDER FORM

Mail your order form to: Baffin Publishing Co.

19918 Epsom Course

Holliswood, NY 11423

Please send _____ copies of *Medical School, Now What?:A Guide to Building a Rewarding Practice*

by Gary D. Steinman, MD, PhD.

I understand that I may return this order for a full refund if in resalable condition – for any reason, no questions asked.

YOUR

NAME_____

YOUR

ADDRESS_____

CITY _____ STATE_____ ZIP _____

COST: $9.95 (by check or money order; no cash or credit)

Price **includes postal mailing** to US addresses.